JANNU RAJEEV NAREN
A. ARAVIND KUMAR
K. SHIVA TEJA

REVISITING AUTOGENOUS DENTIN GRAFTS IN PERIODONTICS

JANNU RAJEEV NAREN
A. ARAVIND KUMAR
K. SHIVA TEJA

REVISITING AUTOGENOUS DENTIN GRAFTS IN PERIODONTICS

DENTIN GRAFTS IN SOCKET PRESERVATION

LAP LAMBERT Academic Publishing

Imprint

Cover image: www.ingimage.com

Publisher:
LAP LAMBERT Academic Publishing
is a trademark of
Dodo Books Indian Ocean Ltd. and OmniScriptum S.R.L publishing group

120 High Road, East Finchley, London, N2 9ED, United Kingdom
Str. Armeneasca 28/1, office 1, Chisinau MD-2012, Republic of Moldova, Europe
Managing Directors: Ieva Konstantinova, Victoria Ursu
info@omniscriptum.com

Printed at: see last page
ISBN: 978-620-2-42503-2

S NO	LIST OF CONTENTS	PAGE NO
1	INTRODUCTION	1-18
2	AIM	19
3	MATERIALS AND METHODS	20-25
4	RESULTS	26-30
5	DISCUSSION	31-41
6	CONCLUSION	42
7	REFERENCES	43-57

The alveolar process is a tooth-dependent tissue that develops in conjunction with the eruption of the teeth. The tooth is anchored to the jaws via the bundle bone into which the periodontal ligament fibres invest[1].

Loss of alveolar bone may be attributed to a variety of factors, such as endodontic pathology, periodontitis, facial trauma and aggressive maneuvers during extractions. Most extractions are done with no regard for maintaining the alveolar ridge. Whether due to caries, trauma or advanced periodontal disease, tooth extraction and subsequent healing of the socket commonly result in osseous deformities of the alveolar ridge, including reduced height and reduced width of the residual ridge[2].This bone loss appears to be progressive and irreversible. It is accelerated in the first 6 months leading to as much as 40% of the alveolar height and 60% of alveolar width loss followed by a gradual modeling and remodeling of the remaining bone[3]

Tallgrendemonstrated 400% higher residual ridge resorption in the mandible compared with the maxilla[4]. Regarding the surfaces most affected by extractions, some classic studies have demonstrated that postextraction alveolar resorption is significantly larger in the buccal aspect in both jaws[5-8]. Resorption rate of the alveolar ridge is faster during the initial 6 months following the extraction[9], and proceeds at an average of 0.5-1.0% per year[10]. The height of a healed socket never reaches the levels seen at the time of extraction, post operatively[11]. Schropp et al.,estimated 2/3rd of the soft and hard tissue changes occur in the first 3 months. They reported a 50% of crestal width loss in a 12-month period, 2/3rd of which occurred in the first 12 weeks[12]. In a long term study, Ashman et al.,reported an alveolar bone shrinkage of 40-60% in height and width within the first 2-3 years[10].

The ultimate aim of implant dentistry is to restore missing or extracted teeth by placing implants in anatomically, esthetically, and long term functional restorative positions. Extraction socket wound healing is characterized by resorption of the alveolar bone at the extraction site.This bone resorption results in esthetic and restorative challenges which reduce the bone volume available for implant placement[13].

Knowledge of the healing process at extraction sites, including bone resorption and remodelling is fundamental to our understanding. Changes occur at molecular, cellular, and tissue levels. Extraction of a tooth commences a cascade of inflammatory reactions. There are 5 different stages in osseous socket healing:

- Stage 1:The initial clot forms almost immediately as a “Coagulum” of red and white blood cells.
- Stage 2:Granulation tissue replaces the clot over a 4 to 5-day period. Angiogenesis begins through cords of endothelial cells and capillary formation.
- Stage 3:Connective tissue (collagen fibers, spindle shaped fibroblasts) gradually replaces granulation tissue over a period of 14 to 16 days.
- Stage 4: Classification of osteoid is apparent, commencing at the base and periphery of the socket by 7 to 10 days. Bone trabeculae almost completely fill the socket by 6 weeks. Maximum osteoblastic activity, seen as a proliferation of cellular and connective tissue elements with osteoblasts laying down osteoid around immature islands of bone, occurs between 4 and 6 weeks after extraction. After 8 weeks, the osteogenic process appears to slow down.

- Stage 5: Complete epithelial closure of the socket is achieved after 4 to 5 weeks. Substantial bone fill occurs between 5 to 10 weeks. By 16 weeks, bone fill is complete, with little evidence of osteogenic activity at this time. Although bone fill in the socket will continue for several months, it does not reach the bone level of the neighbour teeth[14].

Nicholas Caplanis et al.,has proposed a classification system of extraction defect sounding. This classification is divided into 4 types:

Type 1 extraction defect: The EDS-1 is characterized by a pristine, undamaged single- rooted socket, with a thick periodontal biotype in a systemically healthy patient. This defect allows for predictable immediate implant placement in a prosthetically ideal position.[15,16]An atraumatic surgical technique is vital in preparation for immediate implant placement and is a unique and more time-consuming process in contrast to conventional extraction techniques. This involves the use of microsurgical instrumentation such as periotomes and other similar devices and an acute regard to the preservation of tissues during tooth removal. The EDS-1 has four intact bony walls including a crestal buccal plate thickness of 1 mm or more. With the surgical template in position and using the cervical margin of the future restoration as a reference, the gingival margin should be at the level or above the reference point and the alveolar crest should be no more than 3 mm beyond.

Type 2 extraction defect: The EDS-2 is any socket with up to a mild degree of crestal bone damage or interproximal tissue loss of 2 mm, with a thin or thick biotype, a buccal plate thickness of less than 1 mm, or any combination thereof, in a systemically healthy patient. No more than one socket wall is compromised. The EDS-2 includes fenestrations that do not compromise the integrity of the crestal aspect of the buccal plate, such as apical endodontic damage. Another example of an EDS-2 would include an ideal socket as defined by the EDS-1 that has a thin instead of thick biotype. A further example would include a single-rooted bicuspid socket where the distance between the restorative margin of the surgical template and the alveolar crest is greater than 3 mm but no more than 5 mm. All multiple-rooted sockets with any of the above conditions are considered EDS-2.

Type 3 extraction defect: The EDS-3 is broadly defined. It is generally characterized by moderate compromise of the local tissues in a systemically healthy patient. This includes a vertical or transverse hard- and/or soft-tissue loss of 3 to 5 mm, one or two compromised socket walls, a thick or thin periodontal biotype, or any combination thereof. With the surgical template in position and using the cervical margin of the future restoration as a reference, the gingival margin is positioned 3 to 5 mm away from this cervical margin reference point and the crest 6 to 8 mm away. This type of defect does not allow for routine immediate implant placement given the greater risk of recession, implant exposure, implant malpositioning, inadequate initial implant stability, or reduced bone-implant contact. Examples of an EDS-3 defect include any socket with a buccal plate dehiscence of 7 mm from the reference point. Another example would include a tooth with interproximal bone or soft-tissue loss of 4 mm.

Type 4 extraction defect: The EDS-4 is characterized by a severely compromised socket with greater than 5 mm of vertical or transverse loss of hard and/or soft tissue, two or more reduced socket walls in a systemically healthy individual. The periodontal biotype in these situations is either thick or thin. Immediate implant placement in these situations is not possible without compromised implant stability or significant amounts of implant body exposure. Examples of an EDS-4 defect include sites with an extensive history of periodontal pathosis leading to a severely reduced alveolar housing with destruction of the buccal and palatal plates. Another example would include greater than 5 mm of interproximal bone loss between multiple-tooth extraction sockets. With the surgical template in place, the distance between the gingival margin and the restorative cervical margin exceeds 5 mm. The alveolar crest is positioned greater than 8 mm away from this reference point[17].

Nicolas elian et al.,proposed a classification system of extraction sockets. This classification is divided into 3 types:

Type I Socket: The facial soft tissue and buccal plate of bone are at normal levels in relation to the cementoenamel junction of the pre-extracted tooth and remain intact postextraction

Type II Socket: Facial soft tissue is present but the buccal plate is partially missing following extraction of the tooth.

Type III Socket: The facial soft tissue and the buccal plate of bone are both markedly reduced after tooth extraction[18].

Atwood evaluated the resorption process in the postextraction anterior ridge of the edentulous mandible in several clinical and cephalometric studies. Atwood and Coy divided the factors affecting the rate of resorption into four categories: anatomic, metabolic, functional and prosthetic. Anatomic factors included the thickness of the mucosa covering the ridge, the ridge relationship, the depth of the socket, the number of sockets present, the size, shape and density of the ridges. Metabolic factors influence the cellular activity of osteoblasts and osteoclasts by way of nutritional, hormonal, and other metabolic facets. Functional factors involved the intensity, duration, frequency, and direction of forces applied to bone[19].

Loss of ridge height results in prosthetic instability as the crest of the ridge approaches muscle attachments and mobile mucosa. In extreme cases, there may be involvement of the maxillary sinus or nasal cavity, requiring extensive reconstructive surgery for traditional or implant-supported prosthetics. Vital structures, such as the mandibular neuromuscular bundle, may become vulnerable due to exposure and impingement of the overlying denture. In the horizontal plane, bone loss occurs largely at the expense of the buccal or facial bone[20].

Tooth extraction whether traumatic or atraumatic, results in alveolar bone loss both in height and width. An average of 40-60% of original height and width is expected to be lost after extraction, most of which takes place within the first year . This can negatively influence bone volume that is needed for future dental implant placement as well as proper ideal esthetic restoration. The most predictable way to maintain the width, height, and position of the alveolar ridges is preservation at the time of tooth extraction. Preserving the alveolar ridges at the time of tooth extraction helps to minimize difficulties during subsequent implant placement. A site planned for implant placement requires sufficient bone height and width to ensure stability and ideal soft-tissue contours. The minimum amount of bone recommended on the buccal or lingual aspects is 1mm, with at least 2 mm of facial bone required for implants in the esthetic zone[21].

The rate of reduction of residual alveolar ridges is greater in mandibular (0.4mm/year) than in maxillary arches (0.1mm/year). The extent of resorption may be affected by several factors, for example, the number of bony socket walls, bone density, severity of periodontal bone loss, the presence of infection and the absence of adjacent teeth. First attributed to disuse atrophy, it is now apparent that alveolar ridge resorption is a complex process involving structural, functional, and physiologic components. Surgical trauma from tooth extraction induces micro trauma to surrounding bone, which may accelerate bone remodelling. Anatomic features, such as facial morphology, have been suggested to play a role. Age and sex are believed to have an effect on the extent and timing of ridge resorption, with females tending to form knife-edge residual ridges. Systemic conditions such as osteoporosis, renal disease, vascular and endocrine disorders may accelerate alveolar bone loss by altering normal bone physiology and metabolism. Functional forces such as bruxism, complete denture wear, and heavy bite forces have been implicated as contributing factors in accelerated bone loss. Presently, the molecular events in the bone remodeling process are being studied in order to arrive at a more complete understanding of this disorder[20].

Socket preservation is a procedure to preserve soft and hard tissues of the alveolar ridge after extraction. Post-extraction, bone loss occurs rapidly in the initial 6 months as the alveolar process is a tooth dependent structure[22]. A horizontal and vertical dimensional change in the alveolar ridge of an undisturbed socket after tooth extraction is a normal phenomenon that has been extensively studied and reported. These changes become more extensive if the socket's residual alveolar walls are either damaged or missing. Considerable loss in ridge height and width after tooth extraction may compromise implant placement, especially in the esthetic zone[23-26].

Rationale for socket preservation

i. To enable installation and stability of a dental implant.

ii. To reduce loss of alveolar bone volume.

iii. To reduce need for additional bone grafting procedures.

iv. To enable the generated tissues to provide implant osseointegration.

v. To improve the esthetic outcome of the final prosthesis.

vi. To regenerate bone faster allowing earlier implantation and restoration[27].

Indications for socket preservation

1. When an implant is to be placed more than six to eight weeks after tooth extraction.

2. Should be considered in strategically important sites to retain the possibility of an implant option for the patient in the future.

3. Should be considered for aesthetic reasons at pontic sites in conventional fixed prosthodontics[28,29].

Contraindications for socket preservation

- Acute infection
- Where unassisted socket healing is likely to result in good ridge morphology
- When maintaining bone volume is not critical.
- Where surgery is contraindicated by medical issues.
- Unsatisfactory overall body condition of the existence of serious related diseases (especially diabetes, tumors).

- Use of medications (e.g. bisphosphonates, immunosuppressants).
- The negative influence of smoking is identified separately.
- Genetically determined healing changes may be inferred (when different osteoclast activity is known)[28].

Advantages of socket preservation

- Optimal implant position selection option.
- Optimal long-term aesthetic and functional outcome reached after prosthodontic treatment.
- Need of less complex additional bone and/or soft tissue augmentation procedures or reduction of the volume during later dental implant placement procedure[29].

Disadvantages of socket preservation

- Implant placement is possible only around 4-6 months.
- Tooth extraction and additional augmentation procedures are longer, more complex.
- A need for additional measures (instruments, materials).
- Procedures are more technically sensitive. Not enough of saved bone during implantation–need for additional augmentation.
- Further risk of failure of the augmentation procedures remains (inflammatory processes, membrane exposure, graft necrosis).
- During the procedures there is the lack of rigid (keratinized) gums.

- In acute inflammatory processes augmentation is impossible.

- Significantly increased cost of procedures.

MECHANISM OF RIDGE PRESERVATION

Though the exact mechanism has not been fully explained in the literature, the Alveolar bone resorption and socket repair involve a complex cascade of events. Likewise, any successful ridge preservation technique is likely to have multiple mechanisms of action. Based on the current understanding of bone implant interactions, several key concepts emerge for consideration which includes[20].

- Biomechanical stimulation

- Wound isolation and scaffolding effect

- Modification of cellular activity

Biomechanical stimulation in the form of physiologic and bioelectric stimulation of the adjacent bone via attachment and load transmission during normal jaw function and has wound isolation and scaffolding effect by membrane along with modification of cellular activity by bioactive substance evoking a cellular response from the adjacent tissues there by help in bone formation.

The biologic mechanisms that provide a rationale for bone grafting are osteoconduction, osteoinduction, and osteogenesis[30].

Osteoconduction

Occurs when bone graft material serves as a scaffold for new bone growth, which is perpetuated by the native bone. Osteoblasts from the margin of defect that is being grafted, utilize the bone graft material as a framework upon which to spread and generate new bone[30]. In the very least, a bone graft material should be osteoconductive.

Osteoinduction

Involves stimulation of osteoprogenitor cells to differentiate into osteoblasts and then begins formation of new bone. The most widely studied type of osteoinductive cell mediators are Bone Morphogenic Proteins (BMPs)[31]. A bone graft material that is osteoconductive and osteoinductive will not only serve as a scaffold for currently existing osteoblasts but will also trigger formation of new osteoblasts, promoting faster integration of the graft[30].

Osteopromotion

It is the ability of the material to enhance osteoinduction by other substances without actually possessing any osteoinductive property of its own. For example, enamel matrix derivative enhances the osteoinductive effect of demineralized freeze-dried bone allograft (DFDBA), but will not stimulate bone growth alone[30].

Osteogenesis

It occurs when vital osteoblasts originating from bone graft material contributes to the growth of new bone along with bone formation[30].

CLASSIFICATION OF BONE GRAFTS: Grafts are generally classified according to their original source as follows: autograft (oral or extraoral), allograft (DFDBA, FDBA, Puros cancellous), xenograft (bovine or porcine), and alloplasts (hydroxyapatite, calcium phosphate).

1. Humanbone

a) Autografts or autogenous grafts

- Extraoral
- Intraoral

b) Allografts or allogenic grafts

-Fresh frozen bone

-Freeze-dried bone allografts (FDBA)

-Demineralized freeze-dried bone allografts (DFDBA)

2. Bonesubstitutes

a) Xenografts or xenogenic grafts

-Bovine-derived hydroxyapatite

-Coralline calcium carbonate

b) Alloplasts or alloplastic grafts

-Absorbable -Nonabsorbable[31]

According to Ashman, an ideal synthetic bone material should be:

1) Biocompatible

2) Able to serve as a framework for new bone formation

3) Resorbable in the long term and have potential for replacement by host bone

4) Osteogenic, or at least facilitate new bone formation

5) Radiopaque

6) Easy to manipulate clinically

7) Not support the growth of oral pathogens

8) Hydrophilic

9) Available in particulate and molded forms

10) Have surface electrical activity (i.e., be charged negatively)

11)Microporous and provide added strength to the regenerating host bone matrix, and permit biological fixation

12)Readily available

13)Nonallergic

14)Adapt to be effective in a broad range of medical situations (e.g., cancer, trauma and infective bone destroying diseases)

15)Have a surface that is amenable to grafting

16)Act as matrix or vehicle for other materials (e.g., bone protein inducers, antibiotics and steroids)

17)Have high compressive strength[32]

AUTOGENOUS BONE GRAFTS: Autogenous bone is derived from the individual for whom the graft is intended. It has long been considered the gold standard of bone graft materials. Autogenous bone grafts form bone by the processes of osteogenesis, osteoinduction, and osteoconduction. Autografts may be harvested from intraoral or extraoral donor sites.

Autogenous bone is composed of approximately 30% organic and 70% inorganic compounds. Of the organic compounds, 90% to 95% is collagen (type I), and the rest is non collagenous proteins such as osteocalcin, calcitonin, osteopontin and sialoproteins. The inorganic component is composed of calcium phosphate, predominantly in the form of crystalline hydroxyapatite (HA). With transplantation of autogenous bone, bone stimulating growth factors and viable osteogenic cells are brought to the recipient site.[33]

The growth factors comprise bone morphogenetic proteins (BMPs), transforming growth factor β, insulin-like growth factors I and II, platelet- derived growth factor, and fibroblast growth factors A and B. They are mainly present in the bone matrix and are released during resorption of the autografts. The higher the absolute surface area of the autograft, the faster the growth factors are set free. This means that blocks of cancellous bone more readily release growth factors than blocks of compact bone and that particulated autografts demonstrate faster release of bone-stimulating growth factors than bone blocks.[34]

Bone grafting is an age old story for replacement of a missing bone to heal fractures posing significant health risk to patients. Traumatic injuries, tumor resections or periodontal diseases that involve severe bone loss in the oral cavity attract bone grafting. Whether one goes for autograft, allograft, xenograft or alloplast to fill the bony defects, there are their own set of limitations. The requirement of additional surgeries, functional and esthetic problems at the donor site with varying degrees of graft resorption and the limited amount of graft obtained, forced research for an alternative. In order to overcome the relevant shortcomings, numerous substitutions are being tried. Dentin is one such material that can be attempted as a bone graft material. This review paper is an attempt to re-evaluate various studies on different types of demineralized dentin matrix (DDM) that can be used as a bone graft.[35]

DENTIN AND BONE

Apart from the fact that dentin and bone share certain similar biochemical properties (80% hydroxyapatite crystals and 20% type I collagen,[36] it contains some growth factors common to bone viz insulin like growth factor- II (IGF-II), transforming growth factor (TGF-b), bone morphogenic protein (BMP).[37] Dentin also contains variety of proteins that are common to bone viz osteopontin, bone sialoproteins, dentin sialoproteins, osterix, osteocalcin due to which it was considered as an effective alternative bone grafting material.

There are two main types of DDM, autogenous and allogenous DDM. For preparing the dentin derived bone graft, extracted teeth were prepared as described previously.[38] Adult extracted human third molars were obtained and they were then crushed in liquid nitrogen, washed in sodium chloride, 1M (NaCl), demineralized in an acidic medium like acetic acid or hydrochloric acid (pH = 2), then rinsed in cold distilled water and lyophilized to finally get the graft ready to use.[39] Properties of dentin which are comparable to bone:

Osteoinductive Property

As bone and dentin are proven to possess similar pro- perties, several studies have proved that dentin derived bone substitution induces osteoinduction. Yeomans and Urist first evidenced the regenerative property of autogenous DDM. According to Urist, BMP present in DDM and bone are major stimulants that possess osteoinductive properties.[40]Bessho et al successfully isolated BMP from demineralized bone and dentin of extracted teeth from rabbits. Purified BMP is homogenous and induced bone formation in 3 weeks when implanted in the muscle pouches in wistar rats.[41] Although, dentin derived BMP was different from bone derived BMP, the mechanism of action remained the same.[42]

According to Boden et al, LIM (constitutes of Lin11, Isl-1 and Mec3 homeodomain protein) minera-liza- tion protein accelerates the differentiation of undif- ferentiated cells into osteoblasts, hence, induce maturation and bone formation.[43] Wang et al found out that predentin, odontoblasts and the endothelial cells of blood vessels of teeth express LIM.[44] Gomes et al studied the osteo-inductive property of autogenous DDM slices in experi- mental surgical bone defects in rabbits incorporating human amniotic membrane (HAM) with using the guided bone regeneration (GBR) technique. Slices of autogenous DDM induced direct bone formation and were incorporated by the newly formed bone tissue and remodeled. The bone defects healed faster in the autogenous DDM + HAM than HAM group.[45]

Osteoconductive Property of Autogenous DDM

Studies showed that autogenous DDM possessed osteo- conductive properties similar to the one present in bone. Bone morphogenic protein besides acting as an osteoinductive material, it also acts as a scaffold for cells to grow into.

Kim et al evaluated the surface structures and the physicochemical properties of autogenous tooth bone graft material and was compared with a variety of other bone graft materials. The result showed that the pattern associated with autogenous DDM had a low crystalline structure and is similar to the autogenous cortical bone structure.[46]

Carvalho et al investigated the osteopromotive property of autogenous DDM. In this study, he created 5 mm defect in the buccal bone of mandibular molars of 36 rabbits. These rabbits were divided into four groups, control group (defects remained untreated), PTFE group, PTFE + autogenous DDM group and experimental group (autogenous DDM). Postoperatively the experimental group showed normal bone regeneration with minimal inflammation causing no hindrance to bone formation.[47] Nampo et al used extracted teeth as graft material for alveolar repair and concluded that dentin has high affinity and marked osteoconductive effect on jaw bones.[48]

CLINICAL APPLICATION OF AUTOGENOUS DDM

Tooth derived bone substitutes find a lot of clinical applications. Being autogenous, it eliminates the risk of immune reaction. Kim et al used autogenous tooth derived bone graft along with guided tissue regeneration at the time of implant placement. Histomorphometric analysis of the samples during healing period of 3 to 6 months showed new bone formation in 80 to 86% of the area of interest with excellent bone remodeling.[49]

Another retrospective cohort study (Lee and Kim) evaluated the clinical efficacy of autogenous DDM with a mean follow-up period of 31 months. The results showed that the mean peri-implant marginal bone loss after 1 year implant placement was 0.33 ± 0.63 mm which demonstrated remarkable and acceptable healing property.[50]

Tooth Socket Preservation

The residual alveolar bone get resorbed very rapidly immediately after teeth extraction. This causes difficulty in the seating of prosthesis at a later date or might also be esthetically unpleasant. Hence, alveolar bone preservation after teeth extraction is a common practise these days. Gomes et al conducted a human study in 2006 using autogenous DDM. Twenty-seven lower third molar sockets were selected. The experimental sockets were filled with autogenous DDM and were covered with PTFE membrane. After 90 days, the experimental sockets showed bone formation of the same radiopacity as the surrounding bone. Also, these sockets had shown a faster rate of bone formation as compared to the other groups (control group with no material in the socket and the third group with PTFE in the sockets). It was also proven that the experimental socket had a superior bony architecture.[51]

Kim et al used autogenous tooth bone powder and block in a socket immediately after tooth extraction. They reported good healing of the socket after 3 to 3.5 months which was then taken up for implant placement.[52]

The aim of this systematic review is to assess the efficacy of autogenous particulated dentin grafts in socket preservation.

Literature search

A systematic review of the literature was conducted on the Dentin grafts in socket preservation, with a search for articles in the PUBMED search site. In this, a single reviewer selected English language articles published up to 2019, using the keywords “Dentin grafts in socket preservation” and “Dentin as graft material” and “Bone grafts using particulate dentin”. The search strategy was as follows:

1) (("dentin"[MeSH Terms] OR "dentin"[All Fields]) AND ("transplantation"[Subheading] OR "transplantation"[All Fields] OR "grafts"[All Fields] OR "transplants"[MeSH Terms] OR "transplants"[All Fields]) AND socket[All Fields] AND ("preservation, biological"[MeSH Terms] OR ("preservation"[All Fields] AND "biological"[All Fields]) OR "biological preservation"[All Fields] OR "preservation"[All Fields])) AND ("2009/06/20"[PDat] : "2019/06/17"[PDat] AND "humans"[MeSH Terms])

2) (("dentin"[MeSH Terms] OR "dentin"[All Fields]) AND ("transplants"[MeSH Terms] OR "transplants"[All Fields] OR "graft"[All Fields]) AND material[All Fields]) AND ("2009/06/20"[PDat] : "2019/06/17"[PDat] AND "humans"[MeSH Terms])

3) (("bone transplantation"[MeSH Terms] OR ("bone"[All Fields] AND "transplantation"[All Fields]) OR "bone transplantation"[All Fields] OR ("bone"[All Fields] AND "grafts"[All Fields]) OR "bone grafts"[All Fields]) AND particulate[All Fields] AND ("dentin"[MeSH Terms] OR "dentin"[All Fields])) AND ("2009/07/13"[PDat] : "2019/07/10"[PDat])

Inclusion and exclusion criteria

Inclusion criteria:

Randomised controlled trials , prospective/retrospective clinical trials, case reports; studies on healthy individuals, age group > 18 years who underwent extraction followed by socket preservation using autogenous particulated dentin grafts were included in this review, animal studies where the preservation was done using dentin grafts were also included. The language of the studies was English.

Exclusion criteria:

Studies on medically compromised patients and studies on subjects who underwent radiotherapy or chemotherapy were excluded.

Quality assessment

A measurement tool for the critical appraisal tool for systematic reviews that include randomised or non-randomised studies of healthcare interventions, or both (AMSTAR 2)[31] was used. The tool consisted of 16 items (compared with 11 in the original) and had a good face and content validity for measuring the methodological quality of systematic reviews, has simpler response categories than the original AMSTAR,includes a more comprehensive user guide, and has an overall rating based on weaknesses in critical domains.

DENTIN GRAFTS IN SOCKET PRESERVATION:A SYSTEMATIC REVIEW is a **Moderate quality review**

1. Did the research questions and inclusion criteria for the review include the components of PICO? Yes

---

2. Did the report of the review contain an explicit statement that the review methods were established prior to the conduct of the review and did the report justify any significant deviations from the protocol? Yes

---

3. Did the review authors explain their selection of the study designs for inclusion in the review? Yes

---

4. Did the review authors use a comprehensive literature search strategy?
Partial Yes

---

5. Did the review authors perform study selection in duplicate? Yes

---

6. Did the review authors perform data extraction in duplicate? Yes

7. Did the review authors provide a list of excluded studies and justify the exclusions? Yes

8. Did the review authors describe the included studies in adequate detail? Yes

9. Did the review authors use a satisfactory technique for assessing the risk of bias (RoB) in individual studies that were included in the review?

RCT Partial Yes

NRSI Partial Yes

10. Did the review authors report on the sources of funding for the studies included in the review? Yes

11. If meta-analysis was performed did the review authors use appropriate methods for statistical combination of results?

RCT 0

NRSI 0

12. If meta-analysis was performed, did the review authors assess the potential impact of RoB in individual studies on the results of the meta-analysis or other evidence synthesis? 0

13. Did the review authors account for RoB in individual studies when interpreting/ discussing the results of the review? Yes

14. Did the review authors provide a satisfactory explanation for, and discussion of, any heterogeneity observed in the results of the review? Yes

15. If they performed quantitative synthesis did the review authors carry out an adequate investigation of publication bias (small study bias) and discuss its likely impact on the results of the review? 0

---

16. Did the review authors report any potential sources of conflict of interest, including any funding they received for conducting the review? Yes

Study selection

Using the search strategy described above to search in database, 60 articles were identified from PubMed. A search of duplicates revealed a total of 7 which were excluded. After screening by title, keywords and abstract, 46articles were excluded because they used other study design and 7 studies were selected for the review.

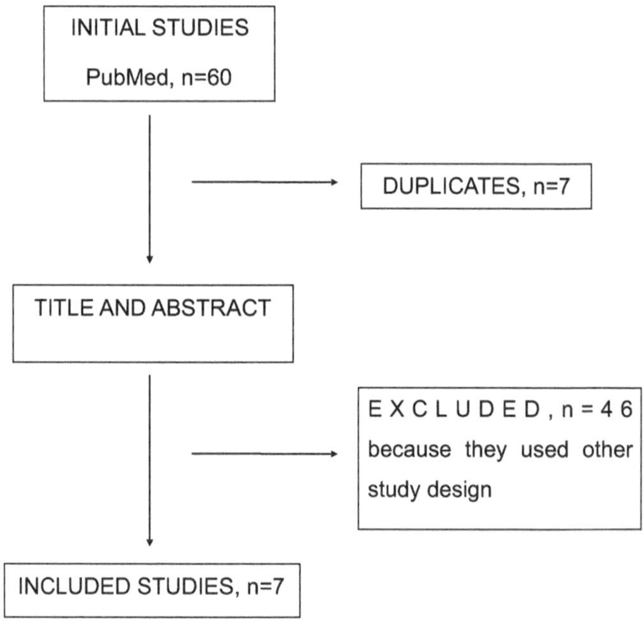

AUTHOR	POPULATION			INTERVENTION	OUTCOME/ CONCLUSION
	n	AGE (yrs)	PROBLEM		
Jose Luis Calvo-Guirado et al.,2018	6	-	Single tooth extraction between maxillary premolars	Atraumatic extraction. **Graft:**particulated dentin graft **Group A:** extraction sockets are filled with autogenous particulated dentin **Group B:** extraction sockets left unfilled	tooth particle graft (both enamel and dentin) can be viewed as a useful autogenous biomaterial for socket preservation due to its similar characteristics to autologous bone. Currently, this graft material can be used in combination with autologous bone debris as an excellent graft material without compromising the capacity for bone regeneration.

GS de Oliveira et al., 2013	16	-	Extraction of upper second molars	Atraumatic extraction. **Graft:** demineralized human dentin matrix **Group** A(left side)**:**extraction sockets were filled with demineralized dentin matrix **Group B**(right side)**:** extraction sockets left unfilled	DHDM induces osteoblast differentiation in implanted sites mediated by BMP-2 and BMP-4, and acts as scaffold for osteoblast differentiation, yielding active new bone formation and may represent an effective bone implant material.

T.minamizato et al., 2017	16	25-73 yrs	Extraction followed by placement of implant	**Graft:**autogenous partially demineralized dentin matrix.	The clinical application of APDDM prepared immediately after tooth extraction to bone augmentation, taking advantage of the relatively short preparation time due to partial demineralization.
Kang-Mi Pang et al., 2016	24	-	-	Atraumatic extraction **Graft:** autogenous tooth graft material, Bio-oss material was used **Group A**:extraction sockets were filled with autogenous tooth bone graft **Group B:**extraction sockets were filled with bio-oss	Autogenous demineralized dentin matrix from extracted tooth grafted to extraction sockets for the augmentation of vertical dimension was as effective as augmentation using anorganic bovine bone. Both groups showed favorable wound healing,

Self Assessment of the systematic review using AMSTAR 2 scale

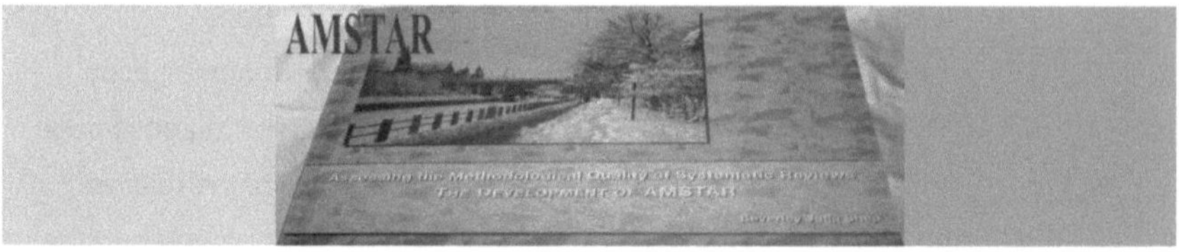

Home **About Us** **Publications** **Checklist** **FAQs** **Contact Us**

AMSTAR 2 Results

Printer Friendly Version

Article Name: DENTIN GRAFTS IN SOCKET PRESERVATION

DENTIN GRAFTS IN SOCKET PRESERVATION is a Moderate quality review

The goal of this systematic review was to determine the efficacy of autogenous particulated dentin grafts in socket preservation. To achieve a predictable esthetic and functional restoration, it is important to preserve the dimension of alveolar ridge width and height after tooth extraction

Tooth extraction is one of the most common dental procedures. Generally, the extraction socket heals uneventfully. However, even with uneventful healing, the alveolar defect that results as a consequence of tooth removal will only become partially restored. Concurrent with bone growth into the socket, there is also well-documented, resorption of the alveolar ridges.[53]

After tooth extraction, the healing process leads to closure of the socket.[6] However, this process is not purely reparative; it involves an unfavorable loss of hard and soft tissues. The first phase of healing consists of blood clot formation. The clot is then replaced by a granulation tissue that, through migration of mesenchymal cells and synthesis of collagen fibers, leads to the formation of a provisional connective tissue. Osteoid matrix is then deposited and starts to mineralize from the deepest portion of the socket. The bone initially formed is an immature woven bone that will be replaced by a lamellar bone. Throughout this process, bone resorption can occur due to the loss of the periodontal ligament.[54] Hence, the overall result of these events is the closure of the socket in association with a dimensional vertical and horizontal loss of the alveolar bone.

The resorption of the alveolar process following tooth extraction in both jaws is significantly greater on the buccal aspect than the lingual or palatal, so that the reduction in width of the maxillary alveolar ridge is greater than the loss of height[6,54,55].The significant loss of tissue contour takes place during the first month after tooth extraction, averaging 3 to 5 mm at 6 months.[12,55,56]

Recent studies in humans have shown the influence of the location and the thickness of the socket walls in the ensuing modelling and remodelling processes after tooth extraction (Ferrus et al. 2010; Januario et al. 2011).Placement of a dental implant in an ideal three dimensional position is critical in achieving a predictable functional and esthetic restoration[57,58]. Unfortunately, healing of an extraction socket involves bone remodeling, which inevitably leads to atrophic changes of the alveolar ridge[59,60]. Atraumatic extraction techniques resulted in significantly less bone resorption than did theclassic extraction technique of moving the tooth laterally with an elevator[61]. Immediate implants may help reduce or even eliminate this resorption. [62] However, there are some advantages to delaying placement of immediate implants by 6 to 8 weeks after extraction: for example, elimination of associated infections[63] and completion of mucosal healing to simplify placement of grafts or membranes.[64,65]

Dentistry has entered an era in which patients no longer need to accept in which their candidacy for tooth must be dismissed because of insufficient alveolar bone volume, height, or width. Bays (1986), Mecall and Rosenfeld (1991) concluded that tooth extraction, either traumatic or atraumatic, results in alveolar bone loss, both in width and height. According to Sevor and Meffert (1992), Grunder et al. (1999) an average of 40% to 60% of original height and width is expected to be lost after tooth extraction, with the greatest loss happening within the first year. This can negatively influence bone volume that is needed for future dental implant placement as well as proper ideal esthetic restoration.[66]

Clinical and cephalometric studies from the 1950s to the 1970s described the resorption process in the postextraction anterior ridge of the edentulous mandible. Atwood divided factors affectingtherate of resorption into 4 categories: anatomic, metabolic, functional and prosthetic.Tallgren[67] demonstrated 400% higher residual ridge resorption in the mandible compared with the maxilla. Regarding the surfaces most affected by extractions, some classic studies have demonstrated that postextraction alveolar resorption is significantly larger in the buccal aspect in both jaws.[5,6,68,69] This can easily be understood if one looks closely at the labial anatomy of the alveolar bone surrounding the upper and lower teeth. The margins of the facial alveoli are thin, mostly cortical (though in rare cases, they contain cancellous bone), knife-edged and frail. When exposed to the trauma caused by extraction maneuvers, the jaw bone is predisposed to resorptive patterns that may lead to unfavourable conditions for implant placement. Commonly, postextraction osseous remodelling also takes place in the presence of dehiscences and fenestrations that magnify the problem, the end result being buccal concavity in the alveolar bone. The degree of residual ridge resorption is closely related to the time since tooth extraction - in both maxilla and mandible.[69,70] The loss of tissue contour is greatest in the early postextraction period (within 6 months).[5,6,58] Apparently, the healing of sockets in the maxilla progresses faster (because of the greater vascular supply) than those in the mandible, which could lead to a faster resorption pattern.[71] Frequently, the resorbed ridge cannot properly accommodate root form dental implants. Decreased dimensions of the ridge may result in the insertion of shorter and narrower implant, which may influence long-term function and stability of the implant supported restoration.[72] Furthermore, it may inhibit the placement of an implant in a prosthetically and esthetically acceptable location.[73] When immediate implant placement is not indicated, socket preservation is a method of choice used to minimize the dimensional changes in soft and hard tissues after tooth extraction. For this purpose, different graft materials and techniques have been introduced.

While there is little doubt regarding the benefits of alveolar ridge preservation, the exact mechanism has not been fully explained in the literature. Alveolar bone resorption and socket repair involve a complex cascade of events. Likewise, any successful ridge preservation technique is likely to have multiple mechanisms of action. Based on the current understanding of bone implant interactions, several key concepts emerge for consideration.

- Biomechanical stimulation: Multiple authors have suggested that the grafting of extraction sites provides physiologic and bioelectric stimulation of the adjacent bone via attachment and load transmission during normal jaw function.[74-76] In case of a conventional prosthesis, compressive, shear, and tensile forces are transmitted to the grafted ridge by direct pressure from the prosthesis. Conceivably, the random orientation of a particulate graft could transmit this load from particle to particle and from particle to bone in a manner similar to the periodontal apparatus of a natural tooth. Elevated remodeling activity in adjacent bone may result from mismatch in elastic modulus between graft material and bone,[77] resulting in increased bone density.

- Wound isolation and scaffolding effect: Bone formation in extraction sites proceeds in an apical to coronal fashion along a dense network of collagen fibers. At 6 weeks, the socket is approximately two thirds filled with new bone.[55,78] Soft tissue proliferation and invagination result in a convex bone defect, with the bone fill somewhat below the level of the alveolar crest. Modeling of the alveolar crest follows, resulting in the high rate of bone loss seen in the first few months following extraction. The principles of guided tissue regeneration appear to be applicable to socket healing. Wound isolation by means of an occlusive membrane has been demonstrated to prevent invagination of the aggressive oral epithelium into the healing socket, favoring the repopulation of the socket with cells with bone regenerating potential and leading to more complete bone fill.[56,79]

- Modification of cellular activity: The implantation of a bioactive substance evokes a cellular response from the adjacent tissues. Whether this response is destructive or reparative in nature depends on the physiochemical, structural, and surface characteristics of the implant. The host response is mediated by molecular cell signaling processes that modulate extracellular or intracellular events. The presence of particulate graft materials may modify the remodeling process by these molecular mechanisms.

In guided bone regeneration 4 methods can be used to increase the rate of bone formation and to augment bone volume: osteoinduction by the use of appropriate growth factors; osteoconduction, where a grafting material serves as a scaffold for new bone growth; distraction osteogenesis, by which a fracture is surgically induced and bone fragments are then slowly pulled apart; finally, guided tissue regeneration, which allows spaces maintained by barrier membranes to be filled with new bone.[58] Utilizing these concepts, it has been proposed guided bone regeneration with nonresorbable and absorbable membranes, several types of bone grafts with or without use of barrier membranes or the addition of mucogingival treatments, and more recently the use of bioactive molecules for the generation of bone in the extraction socket. When analyzing the results of various studies, it should be kept in mind the goal of the additional service that is provided to the patient, which includes the following:

(i) to enable installation and stability of a dental implant

(ii) to reduce loss of alveolar bone volume

(iii) to reduce need for additional bone grafting procedures

(iv) to enable the generated tissues to provide implant osseointegration

(v)to improve the esthetic outcome of the final prosthesis

(vi) to regenerate bone faster allowing earlier implantation and restoration[80]

A number of studies have used guided bone regeneration technique for ridge preservation and reported that the technique can preserve the ridge dimensions more predictably than natural healing does.[81-84] However, using graft materials in extraction sockets can result in remaining nonvital graft particles,[81-87] which may interfere with the normal healing process of sockets in which dental implants have to be inserted.[81-83,88] It is not known whether implants inserted in residual graft particles will show long-term success or not, but most clinicians prefer placing implants into vital bone.[88] Therefore, a material which can preserve ridge dimension and also promote socket fill with vital bone will be the most acceptable one.

Lekovic and coworkers evaluated the clinical effectiveness of a bioabsorbable membrane in preserving alveolar ridges following single-tooth extraction in a split-mouth prospective study. At the 6-month re-entry appointment, they found an average loss of alveolar height and width of 1.50 mm and 4.56 mm, respectively, in the healed sockets.[3]

The choice of the biomaterial is critical for the success of such approaches in bone repair. The ideal scaffold should possess suitable mechanical properties, biocompatibility, biopermeability, three-dimensional structure and ability to promote bone tissue growth.[89,90] Demineralized human dentine matrix is a promising graft material since its organic component corresponds to approximately 20% of dentine weight and is mainly composed by Type I collagen, a bone component. Dentine also contains bioactive molecules as bone morphogenetic proteins which promote differentiation of mesenchymal stem cells into osteoblasts, giving rise to an enhanced bone formation.[36,89,91]

The demineralized dentine particles were chosen to be applied in this study with the intention of exposing the dentine organic matrix, a reservoir of growth factors such as IGF-I and II, TBF-b and BMPs, which induce cell proliferation and chemotaxis of osteogenic cells[92] Considering that collagen fibres are produced by fibroblasts and form a fibril network at the beginning of the healing process[93] and that filling the tooth socket with demineralized human dentine matrix enhances bone formation might be correlated to an enhanced number of BMP-2 and BMP4 immunostained cells.

A network of collagen fibres close to the DHDM, which suggests the degradation of the matrix and consequently the release of growth factors retained into the dentinal matrix. These data are in accordance with results from scanning electron microscopy (SEM) examination of the demineralized dentine surface, which revealed exposed dentinal tubules and loose inter and peritubular dentine fibre bundles, thus providing channels for releasing proteins and growth factors.[94]

DHDM is a unique and absorbable matrix with osteoinductivity properties and the DDM should be an effective graft material, both as a carrier for delivering BMP-2 and as a scaffold for bone-forming cells.[95] DHDM degradation leads to an increasing number of BMP-2 and BMP-4 immunostained cells in sockets at 10 days after implantation. DHDM was exposed to the degradation process and lower levels of osteoblast differentiation were detected. The lower levels of BMP-2 and BMP-4 labelled cells observed within the site of implant since osteoinduction is dose-dependent and directly related to solubility of the implanted material. Demineralized human dentine matrix surrounded and incorporated to the new bone formation matrix deposited by osteoblasts. This is interpreted as biocompatibility of the material, which was reached during the decontamination process prior to the demineralization procedure and the phenomenon named recalcification observed by Catanzaro-Guimar~aes et al.[96]and Goncalves et al.[97]

The effects of DHDM in the healing process of tooth sockets were, at least in part, due to matrix degradation, with consequent controlled delivery of BMP-2 and BMP-4 since the immunoreactivity of both proteins were augmented in tooth sockets treated with DHDM at 10 days when most of DHDM had undergone degradation.

Yeoman and Urist in the year as early as 1967 proved that autogenous DDM possessed regenerative property.[98] Gomes et al had pointed out that autogenous DDM had osteoconductive properties, and produce radiopaque bone.[51,99] Jiang et al have showed that autogenous DDM may prosper in the future endodontic world as an apexification material and as a permanent root canal filling material as well.[100]

Malmgren et al. described the decoronation method. After decoronation, the alveolar ridge was maintained in buccal/palatal direction, and the bone level increased, so maintaining normal alveolar conditions.[101] Pang et al. used autogenous demineralized dentin matrix from extracted teeth to graft extraction sockets and augment the vertical dimension and was found to be as effective as augmentation using an organic bovine bone because of close and direct interaction between mineralized dentin, bone matrix, and the grafted tooth particle material. With no antigenicity, it improves bone remodeling capabilities and can be considered a viable graft option given its autogenous origin and favorable clinical and histological results. Moreover, despite its inductive properties, mineralized dentin integrates into newly formed bone, creating a stable site for dental implant insertion. [102]

Several clinical studies have shown that implant insertion and loading can be performed in both upper and lower jaws as early as 2–4 months after grafting with crushed and demineralized tooth and bone.[40,103] Since mineralized dentin is remodeled very slowly, as compared with cortical bone, the aesthetic and structural integrity of the alveolar ridge is maintained for many years.[49,104] The patient's tooth is comparable to autogenous bone graft material and possesses all the properties of the patient´s bone due to its very similar components to bone, making it very useful in many clinical situations. The teeth and the jaw have a high level of affinity, with similar physical, chemical structures and composition.[102] Kim et al. reported that 90% of the organic component of the tooth are type I collagen, which is very important in bone calcification.[46,104-107] Autogenous demineralized dentin matrix from extracted tooth grafted to extraction sockets for the augmentation of vertical dimension was as effective as augmentation using anorganic bovine bone. Both groups showed favorable wound healing, similar amount of implant stability, and histologically confirmed new bone formation. Thus, the results of this study suggest that autogenous tooth graft material is a viable option for alveolar bone augmentation following dental extraction.[108] It also overcomes patients'rejection of materials derived from animal or synthetic sources,as well as providing excellent biocompatibility without provoking an immune response, foreign material reaction,or infection. Unless it is contaminated by an infectious lesion, a tooth does not cause problems, even when the root tip is left in the alveolar bone. In the present study, the crushed tooth particulate produced more bone regeneration at 90 days than control samples. As the dentin graft maintains the collagen structure, it preserves both the height and width of bone crests.

Autogenous demineralized dentin matrix from extracted tooth (AutoBT) grafted to extraction sockets for the vertical augmentation of alveolar defect exhibited minimal tissue response and bone regenerative potential similar to the much-tested and widely used anorganic bovine bone (Bio-Oss). AutoBTand Bio-Oss-grafted sites showed similar amounts of bone regeneration and initial implant stability at 6-month follow-up. According to current findings, autogenous tooth graft material shows clinical efficacy comparable to that of anorganic bovine bone material.[109]

The non-resorbable biomaterials have great potential in maintaining the dimension of the contour of the ridge by serving as a framework for new bone formation[110] Materials induced an acute short-term inflammatory response with increased leukocyte-endothelial cell interaction, a process often observed after the implantation of biomaterials[111,112]

The demineralized dentinal matrix is highly biocompatible and can support cell growth and proliferation. The particulated dentin of autologous teeth may serve as an alternative to autologous bone for alveolar ridge preservation prior to implant therapy. Dentin graft induces osteoblast differentiation in implanted sites mediated by BMP-2 and BMP-4, and acts as scaffold for osteoblast differentiation yielding active new bone formation and may represent an effective bone implant material.

A tooth is the simplest material be used as a bone substitution material. The dentinal matrix obtained from a tooth has to be demineralized before using as a bone graft material. Being autogenous leads to the absence of antigenicity and enhances the bone-remodeling capabilities. This makes it a safe and effective bonegraft material. Autogenous DDM was further suggested to be an ideal scaffold for stem cells and bone growth factors, and endodontic and tooth restorative material. Therefore, autogenous tooth could be recycled as the innovative biomaterial. Quick in forming bone (6–8 weeks) as compared to the conventional bone graft and considered a boon to the dental world in this era.

1. Van der Weijden F, Dell'Acqua F, Slot DE. Alveolar bone dimensional changes of post-extraction sockets in humans: a systematic review. Journal of clinical periodontology. 2009 Dec;36(12):1048-58.

2. Irinakis T. Rationale for socket preservation after extraction of a single-rooted tooth when planning for future implant placement. Journal of the Canadian Dental Association. 2006 Dec 1;72(10).

3. Lekovic V, Camargo PM, Klokkevold PR, Weinlaender M, Kenney EB, Dimitrijevic B, Nedic M. Preservation of alveolar bone in extraction sockets using bioabsorbable membranes. Journal of periodontology. 1998 Sep 1;69(9):1044-9.

4. Tallgren A. Changes in adult face height due to aging, wear and loss of teeth and prosthetic treatment. Acta Odontol Scand 1957; 15(suppl. 24); 73–122

5. Pietrokovski J, Massler M. Alveolar ridge resorption following tooth extraction. J Prosthet Dent 1967; 17(1):21–7.

6. Johnson K. A study of the dimensional changes occurring in the maxilla following tooth extraction. Aust Dent J 1969; 14(4):241–4.

7. Fickl S, Zuhr O, Wachtel H, Stappert CFJ, Stein JM, Hurzeler MB. Dimensional changes of the alveolar ridge contour after different socket preservation techniques. J Clin Periodontol 2008;35:906–913.

8. Smukler H, Landi L, Setayesh R. Histomorphometric Evaluation of extraction sockets and deficient alveolar ridges treated with allograft and barrier membrane: a pilot study. Int J Oral Maxillofac Imp. 1999;14: 407–416.

9. Pietrokovski J, Massler M. Alveolar ridge resorption following tooth extraction. Journal of Prosthetic Dentistry. 1967 Jan 1;17(1):21-7.

10. Ashman A. Postextraction ridge preservation using a synthetic alloplast. Implant dentistry. 2000;9(2):168-76.

11. Hammerle CH, Araújo MG, Simion M, Osteology Consensus Group 2011. Evidence-based knowledge on the biology and treatment of extraction sockets. Clinical oral implants research. 2012 Feb;23:80-2.

12. Schropp L, Wenzel A, Kostopoulos L, Karring T. Bone healing and soft tissue contour changes following single-tooth extraction: a clinical and radiographic 12-month prospective study. International Journal of Periodontics & Restorative Dentistry. 2003 Aug 1;23(4).

13. Ahmad Kutkut, Sebastiano Andreana et al.Extraction Socket Preservation Graft Before Implant Placement With Calcium Sulfate Hemihydrate and Platelet-Rich Plasma: A Clinical and Histomorphometric Study in Humans . J Periodontol 2012;83: 401-409.

14. Tassos Irinakis. Preserving the socket dimensions with bone grafting in single sites: an esthetic surgical approach when planning delayed implant placement. J of Implant 2007;33(3):156-163

15. Sclar AG. The Bio-Col Technique. In: Soft Tissue and Esthetic Considerations in Implant Therapy. Carol Stream, IL: Quintessence Publishing Co; 2003:75-112.

16. Becker W, Becker B, Polizzi G, Bergstrom C. Autogenous bone grafting of bone defects adjacent to implants placed into immediate extraction sockets in patients: A prospective study. Int J Oral Maxillofac Impl 1994;9:389-396.

17. Elian N, Cho S, Froum S, Smith RB, Tarnow DP. A simplified socket classificationand repair technique. Practical Procedures and Aesthetic Dentistry. 2007 Mar;19(2):99.

18. Tomlin et al. Ridge Preservation for Implant Therapy: a Review of the Literature. The Open Dentistry Journal, 2014, 8, (Suppl 1-M4) 66-76

19. Bartee et al. Extraction site reconstruction for alveolar ridge preservation. part 1: rationale and materials selection. J of Implant 2001;27(4):187-193

20. Luthra K, Aggarwal N, Luthra S. Socket preservation and augmentation in esthetic zone: a case report. Indian J Dent 2012 Mar;1(4):134-137

21. Thakkar DJ, Deshpande NC, Dave DH, Narayankar SD. A comparative evaluation of extraction socket preservation with demineralized freeze-dried bone allograft alone and along with platelet-rich fibrin: A clinical and radiographic study. Contemporary clinical dentistry. 2016 Jul;7(3):371.

22. Araujo MG, Lindhe J. Dimensional ridge alterations following tooth extraction. An experimental study in the dog. Journal of clinical periodontology. 2005 Feb;32(2):212-8.

23. Hurzeler MB, Kohal RJ, Naghshbandl J, Mota LF, Conradt J, Hutmacher D, Caffesse RG. Evaluation of a new bioresorbable barrier to facilitate guided bone regeneration around exposed implant threads: An experimental study in

the monkey. International journal of oral and maxillofacial surgery. 1998 Aug 1;27(4):315-20.

24. Okamoto T, da silvaAO. Histological study on the healing of rat dental sockets after partial removal of the buccal bony plate. The Journal of Nihon University School of Dentistry. 1983;25(3):202-13.

25. Sclar AG. Strategies for management of single-tooth extraction sites in aesthetic implant therapy. Journal of oral and maxillofacial surgery. 2004 Sep 1;62:90-105.

26. Pagni G, Pellegrini G, Giannobile W V, Rasperini1 G. Postextraction Alveolar Ridge Preservation: Biological Basis and Treatments. Int J dent. 2012;2012:1-13

27. Darby I, Chen S, De Poi R. Ridge preservation: what is it and when should it be considered. Australian Dental Journal. 2008;53:1–21

28. Chen S, Buser D. ITI Treatment Guide. Volume 3: Implant placement in postextraction sites. Treatment options. Berlin: Quintessence Publ Co. 2008;11-5(19)30-1,143-52

29. Giannoudis PV, Dinopoulos H, Tsiridis E. Bone substitutes: An update. Injury. 2005;36(Suppl 3):S20–7

30. Mardas, N., Chadha, V. & Donos, N. Alveolar ridge preservation with guided bone regeneration and a synthetic bone substitute or a bovinederived xenograft: a randomized, controlled clinical trial. Clinical Oral Implants Research 2010 Jul;21(7): 688–698.

31. Nasr HF, Aichelmann-Reidy ME, Yukna RA. Bone and bone substitutes. Periodontology. 2000 1999;19:74–86

32. Ashman A. The use of synthetic bone materials in dentistry. Compendium 1992; 13(11):1020;1022,1024–1026.

33. Pallesen L, Schou S, Aaboe M, Hjortinq-Hansen E, Nattestad A, Melsen F. Influence of particle size on the early stages of bone regeneration: A histologic and stereologic study in rabbit calvarium. Int J Oral Maxillofac Implants. 2002;17:498-506

34. Stenderup K, Justesen J, Clausen C, Kassem M. Aging is associated with decreased maximal life span and accelerated senescence of bone marrow stromal cells. Bone 2003;33:919-926.

35. Bhattacharjya C, Gadicherla S, Kamath AT, Smriti K, Pentapati KC. Tooth derived bone graft material. World J Dent. 2016 Jan 1;7(1):32-5.

36. Urist MR, Strates BS. Bone morphogenetic protein. Journal of dental research. 1971 Nov;50(6):1392-406.

37. Smith AJ. Vitality of the dentin-pulp complex in health and disease: growth factors as key mediators. Journal of dental education. 2003 Jun 1;67(6): 678-89.

38. Murata M. Bone and cartilage induction in nude mice by human demineralized dentin matrix. J Hard Tissue Biol. 2003;11:110-4.

39. Murata M. Bone engineering using human demineralized dentin matrix and recombinant human BMP-2. Journal of Hard Tissue Biology. 2005;14(2):80-1.

40. Yeomans JD, Urist MR. Bone induction by decalcified dentine implanted into oral, osseous and muscle tissues. Archives of oral biology. 1967 Aug 1;12(8): 999-IN16.

41. Bessho K, Tagawa T, Murata M. Purification of rabbit bone morphogenetic protein derived from bone, dentin and wound tissue after tooth extraction. J Oral Maxillofac Surg 1990;48:162-169.

42. Bessho K, Tanaka N, Matsumoto J, Tagawa T, Murata M. Human dentin matrix-derived bone morphogenic protein. J Dent Res 1991;70:171-175.

43. Boden SD, Liu Y, Hair GA, et al. LMP-1, a LIM-domain protein, mediates BMP-6 effects on bone formation. Endocrinol 1998; 139:125-134.

44. Wang X, Zhang Q, Chen Z, Zhang L. Immunohistochemical localization of LIM mineralization in pulp-dentin complex of human teeth in normal and pathological condition. J Endod 2008;34:143-147.

45. Gomes MF, dos Anjos MJ, Nogueira TO, Guimarães SA. Histologic evaluation of the osteoinductive property of autogenous demineralized dentin matrix on surgical bone defects in rabbit skulls using human amniotic membrane for guided bone regeneration: Int J Oral Maxillofac Implants 2001;16:563-571.

46. Kim YK, Kim SG, Yun PY, et al. Autogenous teeth used for bone grafting: a comparison to traditional grafting materials. Oral Surg Oral Med Oral Pathol Oral Radiol 2014;117:e39-45.

47. Carvalho VA, Tosello Dde O, Salgado MA, Gomes MF. Histomorphometric analysis of homogenous demineralized dentin matrix as osteopromotive material in rabbit mandibles. Int J Oral Maxillofac Implants 2004;19:679-686.

48. Nampo T, Watahiki J, Enomoto A, et al. A new method for alveolar bone repair using extracted teeth for the graft material. J Periodontol 2010;81:1264-1272.

49. Kim YK, Kim SG, Byeon JH, et al. Development of a novel bone grafting material using autogenous teeth. Oral Surg Oral Med Oral Pathol Oral Radiol Endod 2010;109:496-504.

50. Lee JY, Kim YK. Retrospective cohort study of autogenous tooth bone graft. Oral Biol Res 2012;36:39-43.

51. Gomes MF, Abreu PP, Morosolli AR, Araújo MM, Goulart Md. Densitometric analysis of the autogenous demineralized dentin matrix on the dental socket wound healing process in humans. Braz Oral Res 2006;20:324-330.

52. Kim YK, Kim SG, Kim KW, Um IW. Extraction socket preservation and reconstruction using autogenous tooth bone graft: J Korean Assoc Maxillofac Plast Reconstr Surg 2011;33:264-269.

53. Cardaropoli et al. Preservation of the Postextraction Alveolar Ridge: A Clinical and Histologic Study. Int J Periodontics Restorative Dent 2008;28:469–477

54. Lam RV. Contour changes of the alveolar process following extractions. J Prosthet Dent 1960; 10:25–32.

55. Amler MH. The sequence of tissue regeneration in human extraction wounds. Oral Surg Oral Med Oral Pathol 1969;27: 309–318.

56. Lekovic V, Kennev EB, Weinlaender M, et al. A bone regenerative approach to alveolar ridge maintenance following tooth extraction. Report of 10 cases. J Periodontol 1997 Jun; 68:363–370.

57. Howell TH, Fiorellini J, Jones A, et al. A feasibility study evaluating rhBMP- 2/ absorbable collagen sponge device for local alveolar ridge preservation or augmentation. Int J Periodontics Restorative Dent 1997;17:124–139.

58. Atwood DA. Reduction of residual ridges: A major oral disease entity. J Prosthet Dent 1971;26:266–279.

59. Atwood DA, Coy WA. Clinical, cephalometric, and densitometric study of reduction of residual ridges. J Prosthet Dent 1971;26:280–295.

60. Herrera JM, Steveling H. Alveolarfortsatzresorption nach Zahnentfernung mit zwei unterschiedlichen Extractionsmethoden: Eine vergleiche Studie. Quintessenz 2001;9:863–868.

61. Barzilay I, Graser GN, Iranpour B, Natiella JR. Immediate implantation of pure titanium implant into an extraction socket: Report of a pilot procedure. Int J Oral Maxillofacial Implants 1991;6:277–284.

62. Ibbot CG, Kovach RJ, Carlson-Mann LD. Acute periodontal abscess associated with an immediate implant site in maintenance phase: A case report.Int J Oral Maxillofac Implants 1993;8:699–702.

63. Rosenquist B, Grenthe B. Immediate placement of implants into extraction sockets: Implant survival. Int J Oral Maxillofac Implants 1996;11:205 209.

64. Ettinger RL, Spivey JD, Han DH, Koorbusch GF. Measurement of the interface between bone and immediate endosseous implants: A pilot study in dogs. Int J Oral Maxillofac Implants 1993;8:420–427

65. Atwood DA. Some clinical factors related to rate of resorption of residual ridges 1962. J Prosthet Dent 2001; 86(2):119–25

66. Carreira et al. Bone morphogenetic proteins: facts, challenges, and future perspectives. J Dent Res 2014;93(4):335-345

67. Tallgren A. The continuing reduction of the residual alveolar ridges in complete denture wearers: a mixed-longitudinal study covering 25 years. J Prosthet Dent 1972; 27(2):120– 32.

68. Carlsson GE, Persson G. Morphological changes of the mandible after extraction and wearing of dentures. A longitudinal, clinical, and x-ray cephalometric study covering 5 years. Odontol Revy 1967; 18(1):27–54.

69. Humphries S, Devlin H, Worthington H. A radiographic investigation into bone resorption of mandibular alveolar bone in elderly edentulous adults. J Dent 1989; 17(2):94–6.

70. Ulm C, Solar P, Blahout R, Matejka M, Gruber H. Reduction of the compact and cancellous bone substances of the edentulous mandible caused by resorption. Oral Surg Oral Med Oral Pathol 1992; 74(2):131–6

71. Soehren SE, Van Swol RL. The healing extraction site: a donor area for periodontal grafting material. J Periodontol 1979; 50(3):128–33.

72. Buser D, Dula K, Hirt HP, Schenk RK. Lateral ridge augmentation using autografts and barrier membranes: A clinical study with 40 partially edentulous patients. J Oral Maxillofac Surg 1996;54:420-32.

73. Belser UC, Buser D, Hess D, Schmid B, Bernard JP, Lang NP. Aesthetic implant restorations in partially edentulous patients – A critical appraisal. Periodontol 2000 1998;17:132-50

74. Kalk W, Denissen HW, Kayser AF. Preventive goals in oral implantology. Int Dent J 1993;43:483–491

75. Kalk W, van Rossum GM, van Waas MA. Edentulism and preventive goals in the treatment of mutilated dentition. Int Dent J 1990;40:267–274

76. Ortman LF, Casey DM, Deers M. Bioelectric stimulation and residual ridge resorption. J Prosthet Dent 1992; 67:67–71.

77. Garetto LP, Chen J, Parr JA, Roberts WE. Remodeling dynamics of bone supporting rigidly fixed titanium implants: a histomorphometric comparison in four species including humans. Implant Dent. 1995;4:235–243.

78. Amler MH. Age factor in human alveolar bone repair. J Oral Implantol 1993;19:138–142.

79. Rowe DJ, Leung WW, Del Carlo DL. Osteoclast inhibition by factors from cells associated with regenerative tissue. J Periodontol 1996;67:414–421.

80. Tassos Irinakis et al. Rationale for Socket Preservation after Extraction of a Single- Rooted Tooth when Planning for Future Implant Placement. J Can Dent Assoc 2006; 72(10):917–22

81. Becker W, Becker BE, Caffesse R. A comparison of demineralised freeze-dried bone and autologous bone to induce bone formation in human extraction sockets. J Periodontol 1994;65:1128-33.

82. Becker W, Urist M, Becker BE, Jackson W, Parry DA, Bartold M et al. Clinical and histologic observations of sites implanted with intraoral autologous bone grafts or allografts 15 human case reports. J Periodontol 1996;67:1025-33

83. Becker W, Clokie C, Sennerby L, Urist MR, Becker BE. Histologic findings after implantation and evaluation of different grafting materials and titanium micro screws into extraction sockets: Case reports. J Periodontol 1998;69:414-21.

84. Smukler H, Landi L, Setayesh R. Histomorphometric evaluation of extraction sockets and deficient alveolar ridges treated with allograft and barrier membrane: A pilot study. Int J Oral Maxillofac Implants 1999;14:407-16.

85. Brugnami F, Then PR, Moroi H, Kabani S, Leone CW. GBR in human extraction sockets and ridge defects prior to implant placement: Clinical results and histologic evidence of osteoblastic and osteoclastic activities in DFDBA. Int J Periodontics Restorative Dent 1999;19:259-67.

86. Froum S, Cho SC, Rosenberg E, Rohrer M, Tarnow D. Histological comparison of healing extraction sockets implanted with bioactive glass or demineralized freeze-dried bone allograft: A pilot study. J Periodontol 2002;73:94-102.

87. Artzi Z, Nemcovsky CE. The application of deproteinized bovine bone mineral for ridge preservation prior to implantation. Clinicaland histological observations in a case report. J Periodontol 1998;69:1062-7

88. Vance GS, Greenwell H, Miller RL, Hill M, Johnston H, Scheetz JP. Comparison of an allograft in an experimental putty carrier and a bovine-derived xenograft used in ridge preservation: A clinical and histologic study in humans. Int J Oral MaxillofacImplants 2004;19:491-7

89. Reis-Filho CR, Silva ER, Martins AB, et al. Demineralised human dentin matrix stimulates the expression of VEGF and accelerates the bone repair in tooth sockets of rats. Arch Oral Biol 2012;57:469–476.

90. Dimitriou R, Jones E, McGonagle D, Giannoudis PV. Bone regeneration: current concepts and future directions. BMC Medicine 2011;9:66.

91. Miranda SC, Silva GA, Hell RC, Martins MD, Alves JB, Goes AM. Three-dimensional culture of rat BMMSCs in a porous chitosan-gelatin scaffold: a promising association for bone tissue engineering in oral reconstruction. Arch Oral Biol 2011;56: 1–15.

92. Catanzaro-Guimar~aes SA, Catanzaro Guimar~aes BP, Garcia PB, Alle N. Osteogenic potential of autogenic demineralized dentin implanted in bony defects in dogs. Int J Oral Maxillofac Surg 1986;15:160–169.

93. Mendes RM, Silva GAB, Lima MF, et al. Sodium hyaluronate accelerates the healing process in tooth sockets of rats. Arch Oral Biol 2008;53:1155–1162

94. Guo W, He Y, Zhang X, et al. The use of dentin matrix scaffold and dental follicle cells for dentin regeneration. Biomaterials 2009;30:6708–6723

95. Murata M, Sato D, Hino J, et al. Acid-insoluble human dentin as carrier material for recombinant human BMP-2. J Biomed Mater Res Part A 2012;100A:571–577.

96. Catanzaro-Guimar~aes SA, Catanzaro Guimar~aes BP, Garcia PB, Alle N. Osteogenic potential of autogenic demineralized dentin implanted in bony defects in dogs. Int J Oral Maxillofac Surg 1986;15:160–169.

97. Gonc alves EAL, Pavan AJ, Tavano O, Guimar~aes SAC. Morphogenetic activity of demineralized dentin matrix: a study in dogs. Rev Fac Odontol Bauru 2002;10:51–56.

98. Yeomans JD, Urist MR. Bone induction by decalcified dentine implanted into oral, osseous and muscle tissues. Arch Oral Biol 1967;12:999-1008.

99. Gomes MF, dos Anjos MJ, Nogueira Tde O, Catanzaro Guimarães SA. Autogenous demineralized dentin matrix for tissue engineering applications: radiographic and histomorphometric studies. Int J Oral Maxillofac Implants 2002;17:488-497.

100. Jiang Y, Sun M, Wu D. Clinical studies on apexification with demineralized dentin matrix. West China J Stomatol 2003;21:460-462.

101. Malmgren, B. Ridge preservation/decoronation. J. Endod. 2013, 39, S67–S72.

102. Park, C.H.; Abramson, Z.R.; Taba, M., Jr.; Jin, Q.; Chang, J.; Kreider, J.M.; Goldstein, S.A.; Giannobile, W.V. Three-dimensional micro-computed tomographic imaging of alveolar bone in experimental bone loss or repair. J. Periodontol. 2007, 78, 273–281

103.Huggins,C.;Wiseman,S.;Reddi,A.H.Transformationoffibroblastsbyallogeneic andxenogeneictransplants of demineralized tooth and bone. J. Exp. Med. 1970, 132, 1250–1258.

104.Andersson, L. Dentin xenografts to experimental bone defects in rabbit tibia are ankylosed and undergo osseous replacement. Dent. Traumatol. 2010, 26, 398–402.

105.Kim,S.G.;Yeo,H.H.;Kim,Y.K.Theclinicalstudyofimplantationoftoothashcombin edwithplasterofParis: Long-term follow up study. J. Korean Assoc. Maxillofac. Plast. Reconstr. Surg. 1996, 18, 771–777.

106.Kim, Y.K.; Yeo, H.H.; Park, I.S.; Cho, J.O. The experimental study on the healing process after the inlay implantation of toothash-plaster mixture block. J. Korean Assoc. Maxillofac. Plast. Reconstr. Surg. 1996, 18, 253–260.

107.Kim, Y.K. Bone graft material using teeth. J.Korean Assoc. OralMaxillofac. Surg. 2012, 38, 134–138. [CrossRef] 32. Kim, Y.K. The experimental study of the implantation of toothash and plaster of Paris and guided tissue regeneration using Lyodura. J. Korean Assoc. Oral Maxillofac. Surg. 1996, 22, 297–306.

108.Pang, K.-M.; Um, I.-W.; Kim, Y.-K.; Woo, J.-M.; Kim, S.-M.; Lee, J.-H. Autogenous demineralized dentin matrix from extracted tooth for the augmentation of alveolar bone defect: A prospective randomized clinical trial in comparison with anorganic bovine bone. Clin. Oral Implants Res. 2017, 28, 809–815.

109.Pang K-M, Um I-W, Kim Y-K, Woo J-M, Kim S-M, Lee J-H. Autogenous demineralized dentin matrix from extracted tooth for the augmentation of alveolar bone defect: a prospective randomized clinical trial in comparison with anorganic bovine bone. Clin. Oral Impl. Res. 00, 2016, 1–7

110.Baldini N, De Sanctis M, Ferrari M. Deproteinized bovine bone in periodontal and implant surgery. Dent Mater. 2011;27(1):61–70.

111.Laschke MW, Haufel JM, Thorlacius H, Menger MD. New experimental approach to study host tissue response to surgical mesh materials in vivo. J Biomed Mater Res A. 2005;74(4):696–704.

112.Rucker M, Laschke MW, Junker D, Carvalho C, Tavassol F, Mulhaupt R, Gellrich NC, Menger MD. Vascularization and biocompatibility of scaffolds consisting of different calcium phosphate compounds. J Biomed Mater Res A. 2008;86(4):100211

FSC
www.fsc.org
MIX
Papier | Fördert
gute Waldnutzung
FSC® C083411

Kolibri 360 GmbH
Ferdinand-Jühlke-Straße 7
99095 Erfurt, Deutschland
produktsicherheit@kolibri360.de

Druck:
CPI Druckdienstleistungen GmbH
im Auftrag der
Kolibri 360 GmbH
Ferdinand-Jühlke-Str. 7
99095 Erfurt